10-Day Green Smoothie Cleanse for Weight Loss

Green smoothie recipes to help you lose up to 15 pounds in 10 days

Eric Haynes

Disclaimer notice:

Please note that the information contained within this book is for educational purposes only. Every attempt has been made to provide accurate, current, and trustworthy information. No warranties of any kind are expressed or implied. Readers acknowledge that the author is not engaging in the rendering of medical or professional advice.

Legal notice:

This book is copyright protected. This is only for personal use. You cannot amend, distribute, sell, use, quote, or paraphrase any part of the content within this book without the consent of the author or copyright owner. Legal action will be pursued if this is breached.

Table of Contents

OTHER BOOKS BY ERIC HAYNES

WEIGHT LOSS MASTERY: The Best Mindset, Exercise, Breakfast Smoothie, and Diet Tips on Weight Loss

*****

WATER · DIET · WORKOUT: 97 Proven Tripartite Tips for Natural Weight Loss

*****

Celery Juice Miracle: The Definitive Guide Detailing How Best to Use Celery Juice to Repair Vital Organs, Curb Inflammation, Lose Weight, and Enjoy Healthiness (Juicing for Healthiness Book 1)

*****

Juice Recipes for Weight Loss: Healthy Juice Recipes to Lose Weight, Detoxify, and Stay Healthy (Juicing for Healthiness Book 2)

*****

Alkaline Juicing: Alkaline Juice Detox, Anti-Inflammation, and Weight Loss Recipes (Juicing for Healthiness Book 3)

*****

For other books by Eric Haynes, please visit his Amazon author page.

Chapter 1: Introduction

I want to specifically congratulate you on assuming responsibility for your health by way of deeming it necessary to obtain any useful information needed to take good care of your body. Your determination to provide it with what it requires to stay fit, sickness-free, and energetic will hopefully pay substantial dividends soon!

Contending with weight gain sure proves to be one of the most trying, infuriating, and mentally exhausting episodes one can possibly undergo. Numerous individuals battle with a ceaseless fight to get in shape and enjoy healthiness.

Regardless of the various workout plans, weight-reduction pills and diets claiming to help people experience dramatic weight loss, lots of people the world over (especially in western societies) are still overweight and keep adding more of those pounds every year.

There are several players in the weight loss industry (which is quite understandable, since it is a multi-billion dollar business), yet after purchasing lots of these "Fad Pills" that provide some momentary results, the majority of individuals who get in shape using these trendy diets gain back those weights in three years or less.

You can't shed those excess pounds enduringly by carefully abiding by any unique diet, ingesting a pill, or mechanically sticking to any workout regimen. It is important that you understand that enduring weight loss requires a significant adjustment in your way of life.

You might be wondering what I mean by saying it requires a significant adjustment in your way of life. To begin with, you should discard the idea of dieting your way to losing all your excess weight. A classic diet is set of "food rules" you stick to for a predefined timeframe.

What normally transpires when you end the dieting? All the lost weight comes back!

With the help of this 10-day smoothie cleanse, your sense of taste will become reoriented to yearn for mainly healthy foods thus ridding you of the need to go on any fancy weight-loss diet anymore.

For anyone who intends to lose weight, the first thing such an individual must do is detoxify themselves. If you embark on any weight loss endeavor without first detoxifying your body, then there's very little chance you'll see any worthwhile result. There are numerous variables that influence weight gain, and one major influence that is generally ignored by lots of regimens is excessive toxic buildup.

Basically, people regularly experience problems shedding weight as a result of excessive toxic buildup. The greater the amount of toxic waste you assimilate or are open to daily, the greater the amount of toxic waste being stored in your adipocytes (fatty cells). The moment these toxic wastes get into your adipocytes, the harder it becomes for only a diet regimen to rid you of them. If you're truly serious about losing weight sustainably, then you ought to, before anything else, detoxify your body system. Hence, for a weight loss exercise to be truly successful and lasting, it has to concentrate on both shedding excessive fat and ridding the body of toxins. This will result in holistic better-quality health and fitness.

Chapter 2: Going Green or not Going Green

In the present health-aware world, everyone is continually searching for easy methods of eating healthy. Fresh smoothies happen to be one effective means of achieving that without having to give up taste or sticking to a punishing diet. In actuality, the moment you catch on to it, you'll be impressed by its simplicity.

This is a guidebook to help you navigate the waters of cleansing and weight loss, and I hope you'll find the information contained herein valuable and easy to follow.

You might be pondering within, "It's challenging enough for me to chew up some bits of broccoli in a salad serving; now I have to contend with gulping down an entire glassful of greens?" Quite frankly, it's kind of what green smoothies are made up of. However, refrain from seeing it in that light to help your prospects of coming on top at the end of the detox and weight loss exercise.

Why I want you to readjust your mind is because if continue viewing these greens as those bland vegetables you detest when being used as sides for a dish or put in salads, then you're invariably self-sabotaging the detox and weight loss exercise before you begin. Have a positive mind-change toward green vegetables even as we delve deeper into the qualities that make them ideal candidates for detox and weight loss juicing.

What exactly are Green Smoothies?

To begin with, purge your mind off the thought that a smoothie must be a blend of leafy vegetables before it can be regarded as green smoothie. It isn't just smoothies derived from green vegetables that can be regarded as green smoothies. Once a smoothie bears a green color, it is a green smoothie. It's as simple as that.

Oftentimes you come across individuals asking the difference between juices and smoothies, and trying to find out the better option between the two. There actually is no single correct answer to this question, as both have their pluses and minuses.

The major dissimilarity between both of them is essentially in how they're made. Whereas juicing is carried out in a juicer, smoothies, on the other hand, are made in blenders.

On Blending and Smoothies

On the opposite side, smoothies are made with the help of blenders which puree the fruits and veggies. Unlike in juices, the whole vegetable and fruit is blended together to form a smoothie. Nevertheless, digestion is still faster with smoothies than eating the fruits and vegetables fresh or cooked — since the entire fiber is crushed via the blending process and becomes easier to metabolize by your digestive system.

One advantage smoothies have over juices is that because of the gradual absorption process made possible by the fiber, they do not cause a spike in the level of blood sugar — since they act as a regulator that prevents instant admission into the bloodstream. Presumably this is a valid point to consider if you're hypertensive or diabetic.

The relative ease with which one can whip up a smoothie makes it a superior choice for breakfast and at several moments in the day. Since all the flesh and fiber of fruits vegetables comprise the end product, smoothies are more voluminous than juices — which only comprise the fluid of these plant foods. The key to achieving the finest blend of smoothies is making use of blenders that are top-quality.

Up until this point, we have stated that both juices and smoothies are healthy and nutritious; providing food vital nutrients required for health and vitality. Irrespective of the choice you make between the two, you'll still profit greatly from the vital nutriments contained in either of them.

Correlation between Smoothies and Rapid Weight Loss

A number of people rely on smoothies to assist them in accomplishing rapid weight loss. Smoothie cleanses involve taking freshly-made smoothies prepared by blending vegetables and some fruits for a definite timeframe. The aim of doing this is to cleanse the entire gastrointestinal tract, which is important in facilitating rapid weight loss. This book addresses the right smoothies to take to initiate a proper cleanse for a 10-day period, and other smoothie recipes that treat specific problems.

What's so special about green smoothies that's lacking in others?

Every fruit and vegetable out there can be used to make a smoothie or as an ingredient, so what's special about the green ones that make them the most suitable for weight loss? The fitting response can be gotten from the pigment that creates its greenish color — which is chlorophyll. This chlorophyll, which is usually regarded as a green plant's blood, is what triggers the process by which green plants utilize sunlight to synthesize their food from carbon dioxide and water — a process referred to as photosynthesis.

In simple terms, photosynthesis utilizes sunlight to create food from carbon dioxide and water.

Architecturally, chlorophyll is almost indistinguishable from hemoglobin; which is a red protein in your blood that is in charge of conveying oxygen round the body. The sole distinction between them both is that the dominant atom of hemoglobin is iron, whereas that of chlorophyll is magnesium.

Numerous individuals feel that chlorophyll carries out no different task in green plants than hemoglobin does in humans, thus likening the intake of green smoothies to taking in fresh blood supply. This, though, has no scientific proof.

Chlorophyll replenishes our blood platelets, which then grows the level of oxygen present in our blood. A number of other advantages provided by this incredible green photosynthetic pigment are:

- Facilitation of weight loss
- Shielding of genes from destruction or harm by several cancer-causing agents
- Stimulating faster tissue healing (making injuries heal quicker)
- Boosting energy
- Reducing inflammation in specific illnesses
- Satiation from hunger pangs
- Forestalling of the further development of malignant growth
- Ridding your kidney of stones

- Detoxification of your blood by combating free radicals head-on
- Stabilizing sugar level in the blood
- Treating skin conditions internally
- Ridding your brain of fogginess
- Alkalizes your body to help make it unbearable for infections to flourish

The reason why it's smarter to get your chlorophyll from fresh smoothies as against obtaining it from cooked vegetables is that the heat from cooking reduces the quantity and compromises the quality of the chlorophyll. It isn't difficult to recognize when this occurs since your vegetables will change in color from a rich shade of green to a paler shade. The moment this occurs, the chlorophyll becomes barely valuable.

Chapter 3: Why Green Smoothies?

Fresh green smoothies are gaining popularity among the weight-watching community for all the right reasons! Green smoothies are amazingly easy to make, comprising fresh organic fruits, leafy and non-leafy green vegetables, and water (The prescribed fruit-to-greens ratio is 3:2).

Regardless of their ease, green smoothies offer a huge amount of dietary benefits that lead to a more advantageous way of life. Some of these advantages are weight reduction, improved vitality, satiety, removal of skin blemish, etc.

Ten Benefits of Drinking Green Smoothies

1. It Is Nutrient-Dense. The Ingredients used for smoothies are fresh and hence way more wholesome and nutritious than you'll find in a packaged juice or a cooked meal. The very high heat regularly utilized during cooking damages a significant amount of the food nutrient and therefore compromises the quality.

Green smoothies are packed with gainful phytonutrients and chlorophyll, alongside other properties like fiber, minerals, water, and several other beneficial nutrients.

2. It Triggers Fat Burn. Are you trying to get rid of some excessive weight and become fit? It will please you to find out that green smoothies are a superb means of achieving such a goal. They are moisture-rich and are made up of low calorie vegetables and fruits, which you can consume in great quantity and still not put on weight. Smoothies additionally have a high fiber content that satiates you to prevent excessive eating.

3. It Cleanses (or Detoxifies). Our body normally attempts to take out toxic substances and free radicals, yet excessive exposure to any of them will hinder the body's detoxification efforts. It is important to know that you can help your body in its detoxification efforts by taking fresh green juice. You can and ought to detoxify and purify the body to guarantee you a lengthier and improved quality of life. When your body must have finished using nutrients derived from your regular meals, it must discard the leftover waste and created by digestion activity.

If it fails to dispose of all the leftover waste, food leftover from the digestion activity can accumulate, start decomposing, and release toxic waste inside your body. However, with the help of green smoothies, you can obtain all the detoxification nutrients your body requires to purge and cleanse it of undigested waste and toxic materials.

4. It Makes You Energetic, Glowing, and Healthy. A fit body is lively, brimming with vitality and life. I am certain that eating organically and healthily is the key to internal and external glow. Once you begin eating natural, organic, and fresh foods, it in no time makes you begin to feel healthier and more youthful. So long as your diets are as organic, fresh, and healthy as possible, in no time you'll start bursting with rare energy and a youthful glow regardless of how old you truly are.

As humans, our bodies are designed to feed on diets chiefly comprising fresh vegetables (leafy, cruciferous, plant stem, roots, etc.), nuts, fresh and seeds. When fed with these sorts of organically-grown, zero-processed kinds of food, our bodies thrive and get every of its essential nutrient to ward off toxins and beam with natural goodness and vitality. The moment you begin taking green smoothies, a quick hint that you're back to healthiness will be given to you by your skin; as it will begin to get moisturized and supple.

Good dieting will eliminate some effects of aging from your facial skin, smoothen out some wrinkled areas, blur a number of liver spots, and usher you into another phase of youthfulness. It will eradicate skin break outs make your eyes whiter and your vision better. Droopy eyelids will start clearing out and puffiness will decrease. Internally, your body cells will come to be revived also, making your organs work all the more effectively.

5. It Makes Food Breakdown and Assimilation Easy. Green smoothies are a lot easier to breakdown and assimilate than regular dishes.

That you consume the recommended amount of vegetables and fresh fruits each day doesn't mean you are without doubt taking in all the needed food nutrients essential for your health. There are numerous individuals who their digestive system can't properly breakdown large particles of food, and as a result, very little of the many vitamins and minerals contained in the food are assimilated into the blood stream.

However, because green smoothies have been blended into fine particles, they digest easily. Smoothies take a bit longer than juices to get into the blood; and that's a good thing. The reason it's slower than juice is because the fiber regulates its admission into the blood, which helps to prevent a spike in blood sugar levels.

6. It Enhances Digestion. Our present diet has led to various digestive problems, for example, gastroesophageal reflux disease, indigestion, heartburn, and a host of others.

The origin of most digestive problems is lower-than-normal levels of hydrochloric acid in the digestive system. Once sufficient amounts of hydrochloric acid isn't formed during the digestive process, a great part of the consumed meal passes through our bodies without digesting, producing gas, which causes the stomach to bloat, and alongside some other problems.

The moment these undigested foods begin piling up along the linings of your intestines and begin decomposing, it leads to infection. Oily foods, gluten-rich foods (when taken excessively), trans fat, alongside other harmful fats are the primary causes for these digestion problems. Because the particles of green smoothies are finer than chewed food, it causes very little problems during digestion. This makes most of the vital nutrients get into the body.

7. It keeps you Hydrated. Having adequate water in your body is vital for optimal brain function, better digestion, improved muscle function, and prevents skin breakage. Dehydration can lead to several dangers. Eating inorganic, processed foods, gulping several cans of soda and cups of coffee, and taking alcohol (especially high-percentage alcohols) and smoking all contribute to dehydrating the body.

Most people go through a better part of their day failing to take adequate water due to their being totally engrossed in work. Water is necessary for our bodies to function optimally, stay hydrated, and flush out toxic waste from out system.

Green smoothies aid rehydration of your body as a result of the substantial amount of water present in them.

8. The Taste is Delightful. So long as you add a sweet fruit to green smoothie, the taste of the fruit overshadows that of the vegetables, thus creating a delicious flavor. Several people who disapprove of green smoothies when they first encounter them grow attached a short while after they summon enough courage to try it. Kids relish the taste as well.

9. It's Not Difficult to Prepare. It takes 3-5 minutes to whip up a green smoothie — which is far lesser than the average time it takes to cook a traditional meal. Once all the required ingredients (which are the sweetening fruit(s) and the greens) have been put in a Ziploc bag and refrigerated the night before, all that'll be needed will be to just blend them. The total juicing or blending and cleaning-up takes ten minutes or less.

10. There are Tons and Tons of Recipes. Asides the numerous recipes contained in this book, there are lots of other green smoothie recipes you can lay your hands on all over the internet. Once you get the hang of it, nothing stops you from experimenting a little with some tweaking of existing recipes — the possibilities are indeed endless. Over time, you'll be able to identify favorites and repeat them. But the message I'm trying to pass across is that there abounds endless possibilities in green juicing and smoothie recipes.

There are loads of benefits that green smoothies hold. However, I'll talk some more about them in subsequent chapters. Once you kick start your personal green smoothie cleanse journey, you'll get to find out other benefits on your own.

Best Vegetables for Smoothies and their Benefits

Below is a rundown of the most beneficial green vegetables to use in green smoothies. They have been arranged randomly as this is no numbered ranking.

Arugula: Arugulas are viable sources of folic acid and lots of vitamins, and they give the bones and brains lots of nutrients to keep them healthy. They're a bit spicy in taste.

Beet Greens. The leafy green vegetables of the beet plant have an abundant amount of Vitamin K which helps in bone metabolism and blood clothing. Beet greens also help enhance vision, improve the immune system, and correct dementia.

Bok Choy. This is a cabbage of Chinese origin that is gentle in taste and crunchy. It is brimming with lots of vitamins and calcium, and also possesses anti-oxidation properties.

Swiss Chard. Swiss chard is a leafy green that has red stems, red veins in its leaf, as well as its stems. Its texture is soft, and it has properties to help forestall malignant growths and it also works as a great cleanse for the gastrointestinal tract.

Celery. Along with it being moisture-rich, celery holds a substantial amount of vitamins A, K, and C, in addition to anti-oxidizing elements.

Studies have discovered that the juice from celery improves cardiovascular health by reducing blood pressure, lipid fats, and cholesterol levels in the blood.

It is also anti-inflammatory; as it helps decrease inflammation.

Collard Greens. Collards are green leafy veggies that share a nutrition profile which matches that of kale but are more fibrous and taste less appealing. Collards are a better operator for cohesively attaching to bile acids in the entire gastrointestinal tract, and for that reason are great at reducing cholesterol levels.

Dandelion Greens. On first encounter, you would think they're weeds, but make no mistake; this weed-looking green vegetable is a superb source of vitamin A and K. It facilitates better digestion and possesses laxative properties.

Kale. With a strong and earthy taste, kale is a lightweight leafy green with tough and crunchy leaves. It is rich in Vitamins A, C, and K, and is renowned for reducing susceptibility to ovarian, colon, prostate, and breast cancers.

Lettuce. Perhaps the leafiest and greenest of all leafy green veggies, this ancient Egyptian plant is rich in antioxidants and vitamins. It aids weight loss, is anti-inflammatory, enhances skin, bone, and visual health, and also boosts cognitive ability. Ensure to eat lettuces with darker leaves to obtain the most nutritional benefit. Romaine lettuce particularly is rich in loads of vitamins.

Mustard Greens. Peppery mustard greens are great at reducing the cholesterol levels in the body and give a sufficient amount of iron, niacin, magnesium, and riboflavin. This vegetable plant is also rich in phytonutrients which possess several infection-combating properties.

Parsley. Parsley is a multipurpose herb that is a rich source of nutrients. It is primarily rich in vitamins A, C, and K. It helps improve bone health, regulating blood sugar, is anti-oxidizing, and slows the aging process.

Spinach. This is a darling for lots of green "juiceheads". Spinach is tastes mild (which is in contrast with several other green vegetables). Its dense green leaves truly hold lots of nutrients with lots of calcium, vitamins, and magnesium. Lots of newcomers to green juicing and smoothies begin with spinach due to its mild taste.

Chapter 4: What Is the 10-Day Green Smoothie Cleanse About?

This green smoothie cleanse is a 10-day detoxification exercise comprising green leafy vegetables, fruits, and some water to keep you hydrated. Green smoothies are just as nutritious as they're delicious, and you'll relish the taste. Your body will equally be grateful to you for drinking them. Green smoothies will help you lose weight, boost your vivacity, quell your cravings, declutter your head, and enhance your rate of food digestion and general wellbeing.

Some of the usual health benefits you'll enjoy after the 10-Day Green Smoothie Cleanse include:

- A reduction in weight (majority of people shed as much as 15 pounds of

weight provided they adhere to the guidelines)
- Clarity of thought
- Improved quality of sleep
- Robust energy
- Reduced bloating
- Improved metabolism
- Less cravings

Why Detoxify the Body?

There are numerous elements that aid weight gain, and the most ignored of them all by conventional weight loss diets is the level of toxicity in the body. The moment the body gets overloaded with toxic waste, energy that should be used in metabolizing the calorie buildup in the body is rechanneled towards detoxifying the body, and this then deprives that human body of the energy required to rid itself of those calories. On the other hand, when the body is toxin-free, the energy meant for fat metabolism does just that — it metabolizes the fat!

Basically, conventional weight loss diets usually perform below par since they fail to tackle the body's stockpile of toxins. Getting rid of the calories alone without eradicating the toxins in the body will make any progress in weight loss short-lived. As a rule, always detoxify your body in advance of every weight loss exercise to make certain that your digestive system can optimally breakdown all food inputs without storing lots of it in your adipose tissues as fat.

You might just be wondering; "how does one know there is a toxic overload in their body?" These warning sign below point to the existence of plentiful toxin in the body: constipation, reduced energy levels, mental clutter, weight increase, severe stomach ache, bloating, digestive challenges, etc.

Take this Self-Evaluation Test to determine if you're due for a Detox!

Go through each question and score yourself a point for each question you answer to in the affirmative.

- **Do you hunger for candies, bread, white rice, potatoes, and pasta?**

- **Are you a consumer for processed foods (Microwavable meals, cold cuts, bacon, canned soup, etc.) a few times a week?**

- **Do you consume beverages containing caffeine like energy drinks and coffee two times or more each day?**

- **Do you take diet sodas or make use of non-natural sweeteners no less than once a day?**

- **Is your daily duration of sleep less than the required 8 hours daily?**

- **Is your daily water consumption below the 2-liter requirement by dietitians and health experts?**

- Do you work or live in an environment where the air is impure and filled with smoke?

- Has there been any time you've at taken drugs to combat depression, fight bacterial infections, or other purposes?

- Do you suffer from recurring yeast infection?

- Is there any metallic dental filling in your mouth?

- Do you make use of perfumes and deodorants?

- Do you take inorganically-grown fruits, vegetables, or beef?

- Has there ever been a time you indulged in smoking or lived with a smoker?

- Is your weight above the recommended healthy Body Mass Index (BMI) range of between 18.5 and 24.9?

- Do you reside in a major urban area or in proximity to a busy airport?

- Do you feel worn out, exhausted or drowsy for long stretches of the day?

- Do you experience issues keeping your concentration or focus on something for a considerable period of time?

- Do you pass a lot of gas, get a bloated stomach, or feel unease usually after meals?

- Do you suffer from multiple colds or flu every year?

- Do you struggle with recurrent stuffy nose, sinusitis (inflamed nasal cavity), or runny nose?

- Are there times when you notice your urine is foul-smelling, you have halitosis, or tonsils?

- Have you at any time noticed swelling around your eyes or dark circles below your eyes?

- Do you often treat depression?

- Do you frequently feel nervous, agitated, or strained?

- Do you have skin inflammation, breakouts, or skin rash?

- Is your bowel movement frequent daily?

- Do you experience a sleeping disorder or difficulty getting peaceful rest?

- Is your vision blurry? Or are your eyes scratchy?

Conclusion to the Above Self-Evaluation Test

The greater your points, the greater the possible over accumulation of toxins in your body system and the higher your chances of profiting from a detoxification and cleansing exercise.

For scores that are at least 21, the benefit a detoxification will offer to you will be exceptionally high, thus leading to increased healthiness, weight loss, and energy. For anyone in this score range, I would very much suggest that you take this detoxification exercise seriously.

If your score is somewhere in the range of 6 and 20, then you will possibly benefit from a detox exercise to enhance your energy and health.

If, after taking the evaluation test, your score is less than 6, then you just might be without any toxin — which will imply that your health is robust and you're in great shape. Congratulations!

Even though our bodies are designed to take out these toxins on their own, it's the point at which the body gets overburdened with these toxic substances that it then deposits them in the adipose tissue. Once stored there, these toxins do not disintegrate easily, and this causes the body to be weighed down, therefore growing larger in size. The more they accrue, the greater the symptoms manifest. You find yourself becoming more fatigued, experiencing headaches, bloating, lack of mental clarity, etc.

The 10-Day Green Smoothie Cleanse is indeed a transformative exercise as regards your health. This is how to get it done:

1. Every day you drink up to 8 glasses of green smoothies. What you should simply do is make your whole day's quantity of green smoothies before breakfast, store them in an airtight container, and take them along with you to work, school, etc.

Refrigerate the smoothie as much as you can, and take a third of it every 4 hours for the duration of the day or draw sips whenever you're famished.

2. It's okay to snack up on celery, cucumbers, apples, and other chewy veggies at several times during the course of the day. You can also

take other protein-rich foods such as nuts and seeds.

3. Take no less than 2 liters of water (or 8 glasses) every day alongside some detox teas.

4. Carry out one of the two techniques for cleansing the colon (as stated in chapter 11 of this book).

5. Steer clear of refined sugar, all types of meat or milk; all kinds of cheese, alcohol, refined carbohydrates, caffeinated beverage, foods that have been processed, and all manner of fried foods.

Chapter 5: Questions New Juicers Ask

In case you're just like majority of people venturing into green juicing for the first time, you likely have quite a number of questions on your mind already. There is nothing wrong about that! Just tossing any kind of vegetable into a blender since you heard that it's beneficial to your health is akin to a sprint athlete just dashing about without any real aim. Juicing demands a certain degree of devotion in addition to some financial commitment to work out and as such shouldn't be treated with sloppiness.

Questions New Juicers Ask

Q. Isn't it easier to chew on the fresh vegetables and fruits than going through all that stress of juicing and blending them?

Doesn't this provide my body with the same amount of nutrients?

A. The answer to both questions is no! Two key reasons exist why it's more advantageous to liquidize and gulp down your vegetables rather than chew them raw: the time and the effort factor.

Just take a moment to think about how much time it'll require to finish eating two carrots, 5 kale leaves, 2 celery stalks, one large apple, and ¼ head of cauliflower (I doubt if you'll be enthused about chewing them raw to begin with), then you'll appreciate how much faster it is simply to blend them instead.

Secondly, the above fruit and veggie combination is a sizable amount of food to easily chew up without some burden to your jaws — and doing this 2-3 times daily isn't feasible. However, by juicing them instead, you're taking in all those nutrients in a single rapid, effortlessly-digestible gulp.

Q. Am I restricted to green vegetables alone?

A. Not at all. In spite of the fact that greens should be the main ingredient of your smoothie, you can equally throw in some fruits like kiwi or apple to enhance the taste if your taste buds don't find the regular vegetable taste agreeable. The main prerequisite is for the smoothie to contain some at least 60% greens.

Q. Is it advisable to make a sufficient amount of smoothie before setting off for work/school to serve me the entire day?

A. Consuming your smoothie straightaway is certainly the most ideal approach, since the smoothies begins oxidizing the moment it comes in contact with atmospheric oxygen, thereby compromising the quality.

To solve this problem and retain the freshness and nourishment of your smoothie, endeavor to preserve it in an airtight, non-transparent flask or bottle and fill it right to the brim so it holds the least possible air inside of it. If the prepared smoothie isn't enough to fill it to the brim, you can make use of some fresh-squeezed lemon juice to close up the difference. Asides helping to fill it up, it'll stall any oxidation from taking place. Refrigerate the smoothie until you're prepared to drink it.

Q. Can I squeeze all foods grown from the ground?

A. Some fruits and vegetables are ideal for juices (particularly hard fruits/veggies) while the very delicate ones aren't; however, all fruits and vegetables can be blended to make a smoothie. Delicate fruits, examples of which are avocado, banana, avocados, olives, eggplant, nuts and seeds, are mainly suited for smoothies.

Q. I really dislike the taste of green vegetables but I'm interested in detoxifying myself using green smoothies. Is there

anything I can do to make the taste more agreeable with my palate?

A. Although people who enjoy cauliflower or broccoli sometimes find the thought of gulping down the frightening. You can try throwing in some green apples or grapes to sweeten the taste a bit more. In addition, some moisture-rich vegetables can help to dilute any harsh taste. Therefore, if you're very mindful about the taste, then always have some cucumbers and celeries readily available even if it's not on the recipe to help add some sweetness to the smoothie and lighten the bitter taste considerably.

You can also consider using some herbs like cilantro and basil, along with spices such as cayenne that help add some bit of hotness to the smoothie.

Q: Is a good blender important for this Smoothie Cleanse?

A. We will be discussing a lot more about this subsequently. You need to get a durable and top-quality blender if you want to not only detoxify your body for now, but make juicing a lifestyle (which I would highly recommend).

Q: I took some green smoothies in the past and it gave me stomach cramp. Does that imply that smoothies aren't my thing?

A. No it doesn't! It's actually quite common for people taking green smoothies for the first time to experience some bit of discomfort in their stomach. This is because their bodies are yet to get used to taking in such a high concentration of food nutrient at one go.

What you should do if your body reacts to it, is to go gradually. Blend a little and drink for a while, and when you feel your body is ready for a larger amount, scale it up a bit. Do this until your body gets comfortable metabolizing a glassful or two at one serving. You can also introduce fruits or vegetables that your body is already used to, such as apples, grapes, and cucumber.

Q: Why must I go through the hassle of making a green smoothie? Isn't it simpler and less stressful getting a premade smoothie at my local grocery store?

A. A number of reasons exist why you shouldn't get processed juices or smoothies. To start with, premade, packaged juices have usually been heated during the production process to "kill any bacteria." The issue, though, is that a lot the bacteria contained in fresh vegetables and fruits are helpful to your digestive system and your body. They are usually not the harmful kind — provided the produce was washed properly to rid it of any external bacteria and is organic.

The heating that results from either the large-scale juicing process or the treatment of the smoothie also destroys lots of the nutrients naturally present in fruits and vegetables. Most of the nutrients in vegetables and fruits are enemies of heat, and would die off once heat is applied directly or indirectly to the smoothie.

Also, premade, bottled smoothies contain preservatives — which help to improve their shelf life — and contain additional sugar to help make them sweet and more appealing to the senses. The fruits used in making them are mostly fertilizer-grown; and sometimes, the conditions under which they're made are unhygienic as well. So you're always much better off making your smoothie yourself.

Q: Water is the most important fluid known to man. Why can't I just embark on water fasting and forget about any smoothie cleanse?

A. Granted, water is the most important fluid your body needs. However, when you're cleansing your body with green smoothies, your body isn't just getting the liquid it needs to stay hydrated; it also gets all the chlorophyll in the green plant (which we've learnt is almost as beneficial as our human blood to the body), along with other beneficial food nutrients contained in the fruits and vegetables being blended.

Also, the fiber in smoothies helps to keep you satiated for a while, unlike what's obtainable with water fasting — where you have to suffer through the entire period of the fast.

Q: Is there any reason to limit my consumption of fruit juices?

A. Although fruits are indeed good for your body when taken in small quantities, if you should drink large quantities of fruit-only juices, you're introducing large concentration of sugar (regardless of it being organic) into your blood stream at one time. Such an action can lead to a spike in your blood sugar level, which will eventually lead to haziness or, if continued unchecked, diabetes.

The excessive sugar being introduced into your body can also result in weight addition; which is counter-productive to your aim of detoxification and weight loss.

Chapter 6: How to Prepare Yourself for this Cleanse

Here are a couple of tips to aid an effective smoothie cleanse!

Blender size definitely does have an effect. Make use of a high-speed blender (having a power output of at least 1000 Watts). All the time required to puree your smoothie properly till your smoothie is smooth and buttery.

Nevertheless, if you don't have a high-speed blender and you're not looking to get one soon, make use of your normal blender. All you have to do is increase the blending time to ensure a smooth blend.

Add protein to your smoothie. Additional protein isn't compulsory for this wash down, which is the reason you will see it recorded as discretionary. In any case, it's always a good policy to add a scoop of protein powder for every day for the duration of the smoothie cleanse, since it will help keep you feeling satiated and accelerate your digestion.

The protein can make the smoothie taste a little pale, hence taste the smoothie first without it and afterward add the protein to check whether it is satisfactory to your palate.

Since you'll be staying away from dairy for the duration of the cleanse, ensure the protein powder you're planning to use is plant-based; for instance, brown rice, hemp, or pea protein.

You can also source your extra protein from eggs, seeds (particularly flaxseed, almond and chia seed) and nuts.

Always Chew Before Swallowing Your Smoothies. Endeavor to chew those delicious ground fibers before swallowing them, so it can mix properly with your saliva to cause easier digestion. Thus, as often as you can, chew those pureed greens rather than just swallowing them.

Doing this equally helps you lessen bloating due to excessive gas release.

Know that your Weight Will likely not be Steady. While cleansing, your weight might increase on certain days, while on other days it might decrease. There's nothing to be afraid of here as it is typical. Three things that cause weight changes in the human body: they are fat, water level, and muscle. The smoothie cleanse impacts on all three of them.

Hence, try not to break a sweat if you notice a sudden increase and decrease. The only time you should be a bit worried is when it continues even after the duration of the cleanse.

Additionally, consider getting a good weight scale, like the EatSmart Precision Bathroom Scale. It will reveal not just your weight, but the proportion of fat, water level, and muscle in your body — and this is useful for individuals who exercise.

Take out the stems from your leafy veggies. Numerous greens, like spinach and watercress, are sold in stores without the stems; however if you find them with stems, ensure you take the stems out, since they change the taste a considerably in some cases. Try purchasing them without stems.

Alternate your leafy greens. Every green leafy vegetable has specific kinds of alkaloids which they contain. Actually, these alkaloids are in minute, harmless quantities; however, continuing to use one leafy vegetable for your green juice repeatedly can lead to an accumulation of a single kind of alkaloid and might lead to some health challenges. The best approach to avoiding this is to alternate your leafy vegetables.

You can use collard greens for a week, use kale as the main ingredient for the next week, and use watercress for the week after that. You could also decide to simultaneously use two different leafy vegetables every week.

The objective is to alternate the leafy vegetables often to avoid the alkaloid accumulation discussed earlier. Leafy green vegetables are in abundance to help you with that.

Use more of ripe fruits. For recipes that contain fruits — or in cases where you need to improve the taste of the smoothie — make use of ripe fruits. They are easier to digest since they have live enzymes. Leave partly-ripe fruits to ripen before using for your smoothies.

You can make use of frozen fruits. Frozen fruits are perfect for green smoothies (or any other smoothie actually) and there's no need hesitating to use them. They're less expensive than their fresh counterparts, and contain equivalent food nutrients. They're also the easier of the two to preserve.

Throw in some ice. In order to get a cold and refreshing smoothie when using fresh ingredients, blend some ice together with the ingredients.

Feel free to tweak blends a little to improve taste. There's nothing wrong in modifying the recipes to suit your palate, so long as you don't go overboard with it. Hence don't hesitate to include extra ice or water should you find the smoothie quite thick for your liking.

In addition, you can also add a little stevia to your smoothie.

Stevia is a natural sugar substitute gotten from the leaves of the plant of same name in South America. It is great for weightwatchers because it doesn't stimulate a spike in blood sugar levels.

Extra fruit can also be added to enhance the taste. It is vital to give yourself every moral boost you can to finish the cleanse.

Drink a lot of water. Preferably, drink 64 ounces for every day, as it assists with flushing out poisons. Frequent urination during the course of the cleanse is typical — since the plenty water being taken is cleaning your bowels and passing out the waste as urine.

Take herbal teas. Taking herbal tea helps to improve the effectiveness of your smoothie cleanse. These teas don't just help in quelling hunger pangs — they're detoxifiers in their own right. Great options to choose from are to incorporate are chamomile tea, hibiscus tea, peppermint tea, lemon balm tea, rooibos tea, ginger tea, Echinacea tea, and sage tea

You can always sweeten the tea if you wish.

If your blood sugar is high, make use of fruits low in sugar instead. Anyone that has high blood sugar with diabetes must be cautious of the foods they take not having excessive sugar (natural or not) or carbohydrate.

If you have a higher-than-normal blood sugar level or you're diabetic, stick to fruits that are low in sugar as additions to your green smoothies. Some of these fruits are:

- Strawberries – This, like lots of other berries, is fiber-rich and contains a small amount of sugar
- Raspberries,
- Blackberries
- limes and lemons,
- honeydew melon,
- blueberries
- grapefruits

Ensure you keep track of the sugar level in your blood all through the entire day to be certain it is steady. It is also a great idea to consult your doctor before proceeding with the smoothie detox.

Your bowels ought to be emptied once or more daily. During this cleanse, your bowels ought to move anywhere from once to thrice daily. Your bowels pushing out toxic waste from your body once or a few times daily is important. If you find yourself not feeling any urge to empty your bowel in an entire day, there is a way to induce the urge and it's called a saltwater flush.

Saltwater flushes are used in treating bloating, detoxification of the colon, and constipation during a cleanse. When taken, the saltwater flush helps the colon in purging old fecal material and toxins from the body, and it is harmless generally. You carry this out by drinking a mixture of non-iodized sea salt and water.

As a way of coping better with the taste, first put two teaspoonfuls of sea salt in a glass of water and then drink it. Then repeat this process without delay with 3 more glassfuls of water. Carry this out in the morning before any meal or smoothie drink, and there'll be movement in your bowel in, at most, an hour's time.

Make sure you do not starve yourself. Ensure you snack up whenever hungry but not due for another serving of smoothies. You are on a cleanse diet and not on a long fast. Snack on fruits and vegetables like celery, cucumbers, apples, and other chewy veggies at several times during the course of the day. You can also take other protein-rich foods such as nuts and seeds.

Slow down on the fruit intake. Indeed, they conceal the taste of the greens; however, taking it in excessive quantity will lead to a rise in your blood sugar levels and pain in the head.

56

Alternate between fruits daily. Even though the sugar gotten from fruits is organic (hence, better than refined sugar), it can still cause all sorts of problems for your body.

Stay the course. Realize that when you begin this smoothie cleanse, there'll be an urge to dump it all and quit — there's nothing unusual about that. Nonetheless, it is important to recognize that growth and progress only comes through discomfort. You could end up compromising some days but do your best to carry on. The effect this smoothie cleanse will have on your health will be well worth all the trouble. Try sticking with the cleanse till the entire 10 days is complete and you'll be glad you did!

Get ready to experience some discomfort. Since a smoothie cleanse is something your body is yet to get used to, there would definitely be some initial reaction. You will notice

57

yourself feeling scratchy and hungry. You can turn to some healthy snack options, already suggested, for solace. This will help you eradicate the hunger and some of the irritation.

Nevertheless, avoid snacking excessively, as that would offset some weight loss progress over the 10-day period, thus defeating the purpose of the cleanse.

The human body has the capacity to preserve your expected weight once you achieve it and set your focus on becoming healthy. Over time during the course of the cleanse, your body will crave less food. This smoothie cleanse exercise doubles as a preparatory mechanism that teaches you to eat healthy post-cleanse.

Hence, perform the cleanse, endure the initial discomfort, and enjoy the benefits of a toxin-free and fitter body afterwards. A large number of us eat whenever we're bored. Always make sure you can differentiate between when you're hungry and when you're using food as a coping mechanism to get rid of boredom.

Adhere to all ten recipes designed for the smoothie cleanse. Be sure to adhere to the ten defined recipes as given in the subsequent chapter. The ten-day recipes are intended for detoxification and for weight reduction. These are calculated and well-adjusted recipes containing all the vital nutrients in healthy doses.

Ensure you avoid substituting the water in these recipes liquids of other kinds. For instance, coconut water may well enhance the taste of a smoothie; however, it is equally sugar-rich and wouldn't make a wise substitute for water for someone who's diabetic or a person keen on lowering their blood sugar level.

After the 10-day duration of the cleanse, you can then experiment with whatever fruit, vegetable, oil, nut or seed you find interesting to add.

Remember this: the smoothie cleanse might have ended after the 10-day period, but endeavor to adopt smoothies and juicing as a lifestyle.

Create a smoothie catalog. Each time you make and drink a green smoothie (or any smoothie after the cleanse), note the recipe on an index card and score it on a scale of one to ten (with ten being the highest and one the lowest). Over time, this will help you grow a collection of your most cherished recipes.

Concentrate on becoming healthy and you'll naturally lose weight. If your sole aim of carrying out the smoothie cleanse is for rapid weight reduction, then it means you're absolutely ignoring what's really important! Jumping on a weight scale daily is an exercise in futility. There will be days when you won't lose any weight, and, surprisingly, there'll be days when you'll put on some weight since your body is changing as it detoxes. Therefore, be mentally ready for that.

Ensure you don't spend a lot of time feeling depressed as a result of weight scale readings these 10 days. Majority of people lose 8 to 14 pounds when they're on the complete cleanse diet. Indeed, some people have lost less than that projection; nevertheless, some others have eclipsed that those marks too.

In any case, the emphasis is on good dieting and a healthy lifestyle. Let your goals be long term, as opposed to seeking for fleeting results and then going back to bad eating habits. If you detoxify and follow it up with a healthy lifestyle, you'll likely not suffer any weight problem for life!

What you ought to do is alter your dietary behaviors permanently. This will mean retraining your palate to hunger after healthy dishes. Concentrate on being healthy, and you'll naturally lose weight.

Ready yourself for the side effects of detoxification. It is essential that you comprehend this fully, and I clarify exhaustively what you should anticipate in the following segment.

Chapter 7: The cleanse-proper

DAY 1 Recipe: Apple Blueberry

Ingredients

- ½ cupsful of mesclun greens
- 1 cupful of spinach
- 2 cupsful water
- 1½ cupsful of blueberries
- 1 banana
- 1 apple (cored and cut up)
- 1 pack of stevia (increase quantity to enhance taste if necessary)
- 2 tablespoonsful of ground flaxseeds

Directions:

1. Put leafy green veggies and 2 cupsful of water in pitcher and blend until mix becomes a consistent green.

2. Discontinue blending and put in residual ingredients. Turn on and blend till it purees.

DAY 2 Recipe: Strawberry Mango

Ingredients

- 1½ cupsful of spinach
- 2 cupsful of water
- 1 apple (cored and cut up)
- 1½ cups mangoes
- 1 pack of stevia (increase quantity to enhance taste if necessary)
- 2 cups strawberries (frozen)
- 2 tablespoonsful of ground flaxseeds

Directions:

1. Put leafy green veggie and 2 cupsful of water in pitcher and blend until mix becomes a consistent green.
2. Discontinue blending and put in residual ingredients. Turn on and blend till it purees.

DAY 3 Recipe: Arugula Berry

Ingredients

- 1½ cupsful of Arugula
- 1 cupful of strawberries (frozen)
- 2 cupsful of water
- 1 apple (cored and cut up)
- 1 cupful of mango chunks
- 2 cupsful of seedless grapes
- 1 pack of stevia (increase quantity to enhance taste if necessary)
- 2 tablespoonsful of ground flaxseeds

Directions:

1. Put leafy green veggie and 2 cupsful of water in pitcher and blend until mix becomes a consistent green.
2. Discontinue blending and put in residual ingredients. Turn on and blend till it purees.

DAY 4 Recipe: Spinachy Pina

Ingredients

- 2 cupsful of baby spinach
- 1 cupful of pineapple (cut into chunks)
- 2 cupsful frozen peaches
- 2 bananas
- 1½ packs of stevia (increase quantity to enhance taste if necessary)
- 2 cupsful water
- 2 tablespoonsful of ground flaxseeds

Directions:

1. Put leafy green veggie and 2 cupsful of water in pitcher and blend until mix becomes a consistent green.
2. Discontinue blending and put in residual ingredients. Turn on and blend till it purees.

Day 5 Recipe: Green Goodness

Ingredients

- 1½ cupsful of mesclun greens
- 2 cupsful of water
- 1 banana
- 2 apples (cored and cut up)
- 1 ½ cupsful of frozen strawberries
- 2 packs of stevia (increase quantity to enhance taste if necessary)
- 2 tablespoonsful of ground flaxseeds

Directions:

1. Put leafy green veggies and 2 cupsful of in blender pitcher and blend until mix becomes a consistent green.
2. Discontinue blending and put in residual ingredients. Turn on and blend till it purees.

Day 6: Radiant Green Smoothie

Ingredients

- 2 cupsful of spinach
- 1 kiwi
- 1 cupful of water
- 1 banana
- ¼ cupful of pineapple chunks
- 2 stalks of celery

Directions:

1. Put leafy green veggies and 2 cupsful of in blender pitcher and blend until mix becomes a consistent green.
2. Discontinue blending and put in residual ingredients. Turn on and blend till it purees.

DAY 7 Recipe: Apple Kaley Greens

Ingredients

- 1 cupful of kale
- 1 cupful of spinach
- 2 cupsful of water
- 1 apple (cored and cut up)
- 1 banana
- 1½ cupsful of blueberries (frozen)
- 2 packs of stevia (increase quantity to enhance taste if necessary)
- 2 tablespoonsful of ground chia seeds

Directions:

1. Put leafy green veggies and 2 cupsful of water in pitcher and blend until mix becomes a consistent green.
2. Discontinue blending and put in residual ingredients. Turn on and blend till it purees.

DAY 8 Recipe: Berry Smooth

Ingredients

- 2 handfuls of kale
- 1½ cupsful of frozen mixed berries
- ½ a cupful of spinach
- 2 cupsful of peaches (frozen)
- 2 cupsful of water
- 2 apples (cored and cut up)
- 2 pack of stevia
- 2 tablespoonsful of ground flaxseeds

Directions:

1. Put leafy green veggies and 2 cupsful of water in pitcher and blend until mix becomes a consistent green.
2. Discontinue blending and put in residual ingredients. Turn on and blend till it purees.

DAY 9 Recipe: Mesclun Kale

Ingredients

- 2 handfuls of kale
- ½ a cupful of mesclun greens
- 2 cupsful of water
- 1½ cupsful of peaches
- 2 handfuls of pineapple (cut into chunks)
- 2 packs of stevia (increase quantity to enhance taste if necessary)
- 2 tablespoonsful of ground flaxseeds

Directions:

1. Put leafy green veggies and 2 cupsful of water in pitcher and blend until mix becomes a consistent green.
2. Discontinue blending and put in residual ingredients. Turn on and blend till it purees.

Day 10: Spinach Apple Smoothie

Ingredients

- 2 cupsful of spinach
- 1 banana
- 1 cupful of water
- 1 apple (cored and cut up)
- 1 cupful of pineapple chunks

Directions:

1. Put leafy green veggies and 2 cupsful of in blender pitcher and blend until mix becomes a consistent green.

2. Discontinue blending and put in residual ingredients. Turn on and blend till it purees.

Chapter 8: Green Smoothie Recipes for Various Ailments

Youthfulness

Berry Greens Smoothie

- 1 cupsful of greens
- ½ cupsful of blueberries (preferably frozen)
- ½ cupsful of raspberries
- 1½ cupsful of coconut water

Put leafy greens and water in pitcher and blend until mix becomes a consistent green.

Discontinue blending and put in residual ingredients. Turn on again and blend till it purees.

Watermelon Chia Smoothie

- 1 cupsful of mixed greens
- ½ a cupful of ice

- 4 cupsful of watermelon pieces
- 2 tablespoonsful of chia seeds
- 1 inch ginger

Put leafy greens and water in pitcher and blend until mix becomes a consistent green.

Discontinue blending and put in residual ingredients. Turn on again and blend till it purees.

Blueberry Sunflower Smoothie

- 2 handfuls of greens
- 2 cupsful of water
- ½ a cupful of sunflower seeds
- ½ a cupful of chia seeds
- 1 cupful of blueberries (preferably frozen)
- 5 dried figs
- 3 dates (pitted)

Put leafy greens and water in pitcher and blend until mix becomes a consistent green.

Discontinue blending and put in residual ingredients. Turn on again and blend till it purees.

Looks enhancement (supple Skin and tender hair)

Citrus Greens Smoothie

- 2 cupsful of baby spinach
- 1 orange (peeled and deseeded)
- 1 kiwi (peeled)
- 1 tablespoonful of apple cider vinegar
- 1 pack of stevia

Put leafy greens and water in pitcher and blend until mix becomes a consistent green.

Discontinue blending and put in residual ingredients. Turn on again and blend till it purees.

Celery Banana Smoothie

- 1 cupful of greens
- 2 stems of celery (cut)
- ½ a cupful of water
- 1 pear (deseeded)

- 1 huge apple
- 1 banana
- 2 tablespoonsful of freshly-squeezed lemon juice

Bones and Joints

Lemon Get-up-and-go Smoothie

- 1 cupful of greens
- 1½ cupsful of orange juice (freshly-squeezed)
- 1 cupful of ice
- 1 lemon (skinned)
- 1 tablespoon Methyl Sulfonyl Methane (MSM) powder

Put leafy greens and water in pitcher and blend until mix becomes a consistent green.

Discontinue blending and put in residual ingredients. Turn on again and blend till it purees.

Greenie Pear Smoothie

- 1 cupful of greens
- 1 cupful of water

- 1 pear
- 1 banana (peeled)
- 1 cupful of blueberries

Put leafy greens and water in pitcher and blend until mix becomes a consistent green.

Discontinue blending and put in residual ingredients. Turn on again and blend till it purees.

Green Banana Smoothie

- 1 cupful of greens
- 1 cupful of water
- 1 banana (peeled)
- 1 cupful of strawberries (preferably frozen)
- 1 grapefruit (peeled and deseeded)
- 1 pack of stevia

Put leafy greens and water in pitcher and blend until mix becomes a consistent green.

Discontinue blending and put in residual ingredients. Turn on again and blend till it purees.

Anti-diabetic

Greens Pear Smoothie

- 1 cupful of mesclun greens
- 1 cupful of almond milk
- 1 banana
- 1 pear
- 1 apple (cored)
- 1 teaspoonful of cinnamon

Put leafy greens and water in pitcher and blend until mix becomes a consistent green.

Discontinue blending and put in residual ingredients. Turn on again and blend till it purees.

Flaxseed Greens Smoothie

- 1 cupful of greens
- 1 cupful of water
- 1 frozen banana
- 1½ cupsful of blueberries

- 2 tablespoonsful of ground flaxseeds

Put leafy greens and water in pitcher and blend until mix becomes a consistent green.

Discontinue blending and put in residual ingredients. Turn on again and blend till it purees.

Strawberry Greens Smoothie

- 1 cupful of mixed greens
- 1 cupful of ice
- 1 midsize banana
- 2 cupsful of strawberries
- ½ avocado

Put leafy greens and water in pitcher and blend until mix becomes a consistent green.

Discontinue blending and put in residual ingredients. Turn on again and blend till it purees.

Enlivener

Citrus Pear Smoothie

- 1 cupful of greens
- ½ cupful of ice
- 1 pear (cored and deseeded)
- 2 oranges (skinned and deseeded)
- 1 tablespoonful of flaxseeds (ground)

Put leafy greens and water in pitcher and blend until mix becomes a consistent green.

Discontinue blending and put in residual ingredients. Turn on again and blend till it purees.

Coco Berry Smoothie

- 1 cupful of greens
- 1 cupful of water
- 2 peaches (skinned and deseeded)
- 1 banana (preferably frozen)
- ½ a cupful of wolfberries

- ½ a cupful of coconut flesh (diced)

Put leafy greens and water in pitcher and blend until mix becomes a consistent green.

Discontinue blending and put in residual ingredients. Turn on again and blend till it purees.

Cardiovascular health

Almond Cinnamon Smoothie

- 1 cupful of mesclun greens
- 1½ cupsful of almond milk
- 2 bananas
- ½ a teaspoonful of cinnamon

Put leafy greens and water in pitcher and blend until mix becomes a consistent green.

Discontinue blending and put in residual ingredients. Turn on again and blend till it purees.

Oily Citrus Smoothie

- 1 cupful of baby spinach
- 1 cupful of water
- 2 oranges (peeled and deseeded)
- 1 cupful of red grapes
- 2 tablespoonsful of ground flaxseeds
- 2 tablespoonsful of sunflower oil

Put leafy greens and water in pitcher and blend until mix becomes a consistent green.

Discontinue blending and put in residual ingredients. Turn on again and blend till it purees.

Avocado Berry Smoothie

- 1 cupful of arugula
- 1 cupful of water
- 1½ cupsful of peaches (preferably frozen)
- 1 cupful of fresh mixed berries
- 1 small avocado (peeled and pitted)

Put leafy greens and water in pitcher and blend until mix becomes a consistent green.

Discontinue blending and put in residual ingredients. Turn on again and blend till it purees.

Immunity Enhancer

Greenie Strawberry Smoothie

- 1 cupful of mixed greens
- Juice of one lemon (freshly-squeezed)
- ½ a cupful of frozen strawberries
- 1 banana
- 1 pack of stevia

Put leafy greens and water in pitcher and blend until mix becomes a consistent green.

Discontinue blending and put in residual ingredients. Turn on again and blend till it purees.

Mango Berry Smoothie

- 1 cupful of mesclun greens
- 1 cupful of water
- ½ a cupful of frozen blackberries
- 1 orange (skinned and deseeded
- ½ a cupful of frozen raspberries

- 1 pack of stevia
- 1 cupful of frozen mango chunks

Put leafy greens and water in pitcher and blend until mix becomes a consistent green.

Discontinue blending and put in residual ingredients. Turn on again and blend till it purees.

Baby-Friendly

Flaxy Banana Smoothie

- 1 cupful of mesclun greens
- 1 cupful of water
- 1 banana
- 1½ a cupsful of frozen blueberries
- ½ a cupful of ground flaxseeds
- 1 pack of stevia

Put leafy greens and water in pitcher and blend until mix becomes a consistent green.

Discontinue blending and put in residual ingredients. Turn on again and blend till it purees.

Berry Greens Smoothie

- ½ a cupful of greens
- 2 cupsful of coconut milk
- 1 banana (peeled and frozen)
- ½ a cupful of blueberries (frozen)

- 3 dates (pitted)
- 1 a cupful of blackberries (frozen)

Put leafy greens and water in pitcher and blend until mix becomes a consistent green.

Discontinue blending and put in residual ingredients. Turn on again and blend till it purees.

Cheer-You-Up Smoothies

Greasy Mango Smoothie

- 1 cupful of greens
- 1½ cupsful of almond/coconut milk
- 1½ cupsful of mango chunks (frozen)
- 1 banana
- 1 tablespoonful of extra-light olive oil

Put leafy greens and water in pitcher and blend until mix becomes a consistent green.

Discontinue blending and put in residual ingredients. Turn on again and blend till it purees.

Berry Pastiche Smoothie

- 1 cupsful of mixed greens
- 1½ cupsful of water
- 1 banana
- 2 cupsful of mixed berries (frozen)
- 2 tablespoonsful of flaxseed (ground)

Put leafy greens and water in pitcher and blend until mix becomes a consistent green.

Discontinue blending and put in residual ingredients. Turn on again and blend till it purees.

Citrus Avocado Smoothie

- 1 cupful of Arugula
- ½ a cupful of ice
- 2 oranges (peeled and deseeded)
- 1 banana
- ½ an avocado

Put leafy greens and water in pitcher and blend until mix becomes a consistent green.

Discontinue blending and put in residual ingredients. Turn on again and blend till it purees.

Fat Burner

Citrus Banana Smoothie

- 1 cupful of spinach
- ½ a cupful of water
- 2 oranges
- 2 bananas

Put leafy greens and water in pitcher and blend until mix becomes a consistent green.

Discontinue blending and put in residual ingredients. Turn on again and blend till it purees.

Berry Melon Smoothie

- 2 bunches greens
- 1 cup water
- ½ melon, stripped and seeded
- 1½ cups solidified strawberries

Put leafy greens and water in pitcher and blend until mix becomes a consistent green.

Discontinue blending and put in residual ingredients. Turn on again and blend till it purees.

Peachy Berry Smoothie

- 1 cupful of mesclun greens
- 1 cupful of water
- 1½ cupsful of peaches (frozen)
- 1 cupful of strawberries (frozen)

Put leafy greens and water in pitcher and blend until mix becomes a consistent green.

Discontinue blending and put in residual ingredients. Turn on again and blend till it purees.

Banana Chia Greens Smoothie

- 2 handfuls of greens
- 2 cupsful of water
- 1 banana

- 3 pears
- 2 tablespoonsful of chia seeds (ground)

Put leafy greens and water in pitcher and blend until mix becomes a consistent green.

Discontinue blending and put in residual ingredients. Turn on again and blend till it purees.

Pineapple Citrus Smoothie

- 1 cupful of mesclun greens
- 1 cupful of ice
- 1 cupful of pineapple cuts
- 2 oranges

Put leafy greens and water in pitcher and blend until mix becomes a consistent green.

Discontinue blending and put in residual ingredients. Turn on again and blend till it purees.

Flaxseed Watermelon Smoothie

- 1 cupful of mixed greens
- 1 cupful of ice
- 2 cupsful of watermelon
- 1 teaspoonful of ground flaxseed

Put leafy greens and water in pitcher and blend until mix becomes a consistent green.

Discontinue blending and put in residual ingredients. Turn on again and blend till it purees.

Grapefruit Coconut Smoothie

- 2 handfuls of spinach
- ½ cup ice
- 1 cupful of pineapple chunks
- 1 pink grapefruit

Put leafy greens and water in pitcher and blend until mix becomes a consistent green.

Discontinue blending and put in residual ingredients. Turn on again and blend till it purees.

Conclusion

All through the pages of this book we have studied about what green smoothies are and how they can be used to detoxify the body and to help it lose weight.

Green smoothies are great for your health and for fostering weight loss post-cleanse. Majority of people don't consume anything close to the recommended daily fruits and vegetables requirement, and smoothies are helpful in making up for that nutritional gap. Green smoothies, when done properly with leafy greens, fruits, stem and root vegetables to provide your body all it requires to remain in health and vitality.

Just to go over the vital things we've discussed, here's a recap:

- Make use of only fresh organic fruits and vegetable as often as you can.

- Always wash fruits and vegetables properly before every use.
- Whenever possible, consume your smoothies as soon as you're done blending.
- Eliminate activities detrimental to your health, like smoking, taking alcohol, caffeine, or excessive amounts of sugar no less than two weeks before you begin the cleanse (and even after the cleanse, the lesser the quantity of these you take, the better).

At this point, you already have all the information you need to begin the smoothie cleanse, it's now time for action! Please follow the guidelines and recipes in this book to help you achieve the best results.

Starting is the hardest thing to do; but once you begin, you can only get better from then on. Take control of your health, and watch as the dividends begin to come rewardingly.

Thanks once again for making out time to go through this, and happy detoxing!

Other Books by Eric Haynes

WEIGHT LOSS MASTERY: The Best
Mindset, Exercise, Breakfast Smoothie, and
Diet Tips on Weight Loss

*****

WATER · DIET · WORKOUT: 97 Proven
Tripartite Tips for Natural Weight Loss

*****

Celery Juice Miracle: The Definitive Guide
Detailing How Best to Use Celery Juice to
Repair Vital Organs, Curb Inflammation, Lose
Weight, and Enjoy Healthiness (Juicing for
Healthiness Book 1)

*****

Juice Recipes for Weight Loss: Healthy Juice
Recipes to Lose Weight, Detoxify, and Stay
Healthy (Juicing for Healthiness Book 2)

*****

<u>Alkaline Juicing: Alkaline Juice Detox, Anti-Inflammation, and Weight Loss Recipes (Juicing for Healthiness Book 3)</u>

*****

For other books by Eric Haynes, please visit his Amazon author page.

Index

C

G

T

V